THE GOOD MENOPAUSE DIET

An ultimate guide to balancing hormones for optimum health in menopause

Vanessa D, Daniel

Table of contents

Chapter 1

The Truth About Menopause

The last or final menstrual period is referred to as the menopause. A woman is regarded as postmenopausal when she has gone 12 months without ovulating. Circular production of oestrogen and progesterone stops during menopause due to lack of ovarian follicles, follicular development, and ovulation. The average age of onset for menopause in women is 51 years old, and it typically occurs between the ages of 45 and 55.

The term "surgical menopause" describes menopause brought on by a bilateral oophorectomy. Early menopause or premature ovarian insufficiency can happen before the age of 40 as a result of natural ovarian decline, ovarian removal surgery, or chemotherapy/radiotherapy.

When menopause starts between the ages of 40 and 45, it is said to be "early." sheets Chemotherapy and radiation treatment caused an early menopause. Considering that women now live for around a third of their lives beyond menopause, it's more crucial than ever to maintain good physical and mental health at this time. Menopause naturally occurs without any sort of medical or surgical intervention. It moves slowly over three stages:
Perimenopause
Perimenopause. When your ovaries gradually start producing less estrogen, this period often starts many years before menopause. Up until menopause, when your ovaries cease producing eggs, you are in perimenopause. Estrogen levels decline more quickly in the latter one to two years of

this period. Symptoms of menopause are common among women.

Menopause.
Postmenopause menopause is seen as "early" menopause. After menopause, these are the years. Hot flashes and other menopausal VMS often subside. However, as you age, the health concerns associated with the decrease of estrogen rise.
perimenopause defined.
The perimenopause, which lasts from one year before the menopause to the time immediately after it, is characterized by hormonal volatility, anovulatory cycles, the beginning of irregular menstrual cycles, and symptoms. The interval preceding the last menstrual cycle is known as the menopausal transition. Changes in a woman's menstrual cycle, such as irregular periods or variations in flow, are hallmarks of the perimenopause. Cycles can have a variety of lengths.
Aside from aches and pains, hot flashes and night sweats, weariness or irritability may

also be symptoms. such as sore breasts. Contraception is necessary because pregnancy can happen despite irregular menstrual periods and anovulation in certain women. Before their last menstruation, some women may have menopausal symptoms for five to ten years. It is impossible to anticipate when menopause symptoms may begin in a woman or how long they will remain.
Menopause symptoms and physical changes.

When oestrogen production ceases naturally during menopause, there may be a "raging" of consequences, ranging from uncomfortable to pathological. Only 20% of women say they have no symptoms of menopause.
Hot flushes, night sweats, trouble sleeping, body aches and pains, dry skin, vaginal dryness, loss of libido, frequent urination, and mood and cognitive problems are typical symptoms that peri- and

postmenopausal women frequently describe. Some females may experience skin changes, pubic hair loss, itching, and unwanted hair growth. Menopausal symptoms are influenced by a variety of biopsychosocial variables, such as the cause of menopause, the woman's age, her physical and mental health, her attitude toward menopause, her ethnicity, and her level of education.

Vasomotor signs (hot flushes and sweats)
Menopause symptoms, which include hot flashes and night sweats, are common in 75% of postmenopausal women, with 25% of them experiencing severe symptoms. Different nations and ethnic groups have different percentages of women reporting hot flushes. Although the typical length of symptoms is 7, they might go away in 2 to 5 years.
A hot flush is a condition in which a person experiences intense heat, which is accompanied by objective symptoms of

cutaneous vasodilation and a resulting reduction in body temperature. A woman's thermoneutral zone is smaller when she lacks estrogen. Despite a little rise in core body temperature, they experience intense heat. Sweating and peripheral vasodilation promote heat loss.

Recent research demonstrates postmenopausal women's enlargement of KNDY neurons in the hypothalamus. These neurons produce Neurokinin B, which is thought to cause flushes of heat. Vasomotor instability in the menopause, which has a negative impact on quality of life, relationships, employment, and wellness, is a key contributing factor to disturbed sleep throughout the menopause. Vasomotor symptoms can potentially be a sign of cardiovascular illness, with more severe symptoms and earlier start having more significance.

Menopause-related genitourinary syndrome

Menopausal urogenital symptoms, also known as vulvovaginal atrophy or genitourinary syndrome of menopause, are frequent but frequently "suffered in silence" since women may be unwilling to admit these symptoms. Vaginal dryness, burning, irritation, reduced lubrication during sexual activity, dyspareunia, and a higher risk of urethral infections are among the symptoms. pubic hair thinning, loss of the labial fat pad, Oestrogen depletion in the menopause results in decreased vaginal calibre and changes in the vaginal mucosa. When vasomotor symptoms have subsided, elderly women typically continue to experience these sensations.

Menopause-related psychological and cognitive symptoms
Changes in mood, anxiety, impatience, and forgetfulness can be caused by hormonal changes, vasomotor symptoms, and lack of sleep. These factors might also make it difficult to concentrate or make decisions.

Women frequently lament having "brain fog" or "brain fade." Serotonin, a neurotransmitter that controls mood, emotions, and sleep, decreases by 50% during menopause when oestrogen levels fall.

Although depression is not more prevalent at the menopause than at other life phases, a woman may be more susceptible due to stress during the peri-menopause and a history of depression, particularly post-natal depression.

Skin Alterations

Menopause is linked to dry skin because oestrogen boosts the formation of glycosaminoglycans, encourages the creation of sebum, increases water retention, and enhances stratum corneum barrier function. Elastin degradation, a decrease in microvasculature, and epidermal thinning also take place. Axillary and pubic hair are less abundant. While some women experience itching, others describe feeling ants crawling across their skin.

 Bone and muscle

In postmenopausal women, aging and menopause both affect how strong and how much muscle they have. A decrease in estrogen levels is linked to the menopausal transition. estrogen, growth hormone, IGF-1, DHEA, a reduction in the synthesis of muscle proteins, and an upsurge in inflammation. However, in postmenopausal women, inadequate physical activity, low protein consumption (0.8 g/kg/day), and high oxidative stress are the main causes of sarcopenia.

Low bone mass and micro architectural degeneration of bone tissue, which increases bone fragility and, as a result, the risk of fracture, are the hallmarks of osteoporosis, a systemic skeletal disease. Estrogen inhibits excessive osteoclastic resorption, reduces bone loss, and may even rebuild damaged bone. As a result, postmenopausal women are more likely to develop osteoporosis and one in three women over the age of 50 will have a fragility fracture.

The fourth most common cause of chronic illness and morbidity is fragility fractures. There are mortality rates of up to 25% that happen within the first year following a hip fracture. A clinical osteoporosis risk assessment should be performed on all postmenopausal women.

Changes in metabolism

Aging and the decline in estrogen that comes with menopause create metabolic changes that raise the risk of cardiovascular disease, the primary killer of women. Atherosclerosis is characterized by an increase in visceral fat, unfavorable lipid and blood vessel alterations, endothelial dysfunction, increased insulin resistance, elevated blood pressure, and activation of the renin-angiotensin system.

How to identify menopause

Menopause is a clinical diagnosis given to women over 45 based on their symptoms and menstrual cycle alterations. Where a lady has had her ovaries surgically removed, the diagnosis is clear. FSH testing is not recommended for perimenopause or menopause diagnosis. Given that women's hormone levels might vary from day to day, a single hormone test, such as a measurement of high follicle-stimulating hormone (FSH), is not a reliable sign of perimenopause. Investigations could be necessary, though, in some circumstances, such as if the woman has undergone a hysterectomy; if there is suspicion that the symptoms may be caused by an illness (such as a thyroid condition rather than aging naturally); or if the woman is under 45 years old.

How should the signs be treated?
Menopause management calls for a thorough assessment of symptoms, risk of chronic illness, lifestyle, and proper

screening, as well as the creation of an individualized strategy that takes into account the woman's treatment objectives and a risk: benefit analysis. Menopausal hormone therapy, non-hormonal contraception, non-pharmacological contraception, and lifestyle changes are some of the available management choices.

Positivity toward the menopause
Menopause may cause physical and mental changes in women, but that doesn't imply things have become worse! This is the moment when many women feel the need to "take stock" of their life and establish new objectives.

Many women may be balancing their jobs as moms of adolescents, caregivers of aging parents, and employees throughout menopause. According to experts, it's crucial to schedule some "me time" to keep your life balanced. Menopause may be viewed as a fresh start; it's a good time to evaluate one's lifestyle and health and to resolve to work toward maintaining health as one age.

Chapter 2

Changes In Hormones During Menopause

All women eventually experience menopause, but many don't give it any thought until it actually happens. It represents a turning point in many women's lives and is accompanied by a variety of symptoms brought on by shifting hormone levels. Let's first establish what the term "menopause" means before looking at the main hormones that fluctuate throughout the menopause in this article.

Due to diminishing levels of oestrogen, progesterone, and testosterone and an increase in the control hormones FSH and LH, women who are entering and transitioning through menopause will have hormonal imbalance.

During the perimenopause, these hormonal shifts will have varied degrees of negative effects on a woman's physical and mental health, resulting in a variety of symptoms.

The perimenopause, often known as the time right before menopause, is a time when women's hormones alter. Their physical, mental, and emotional wellbeing may be impacted to varied degrees. When describing how they are feeling, women will occasionally say, "I'm feeling hormonal," but for many who are beginning the menopausal transition, this mood can swiftly become a reality.

Associated hormones with menopause

Numerous hormones are active during the menopause, and each one is important in causing both physical and psychological change.Oestrogen, progesterone, and testosterone are the major hormones, although additional hormones including the regulators follicle-stimulating hormone

(FSH) and luteinizing hormone (LH) also play a role.

Less oestrogen and progesterone are produced by the ovaries as women approach menopause. The brain's pituitary gland releases the control hormones FSH and LH, which cause the ovaries to become less receptive to, leading to increased levels of these control hormones.

The three primary hormones—oestrogen, progesterone, and testosterone—as well as their functions during the menopause are examined.

Estrogen

Types Of Estrogen

One of the two primary sex hormones in women, along with progesterone, estrogen is mostly generated in the ovaries. However, minor quantities are also produced in the adrenal glands.The primary oestrogen during pregnancy is oestriol, and the only oestrogen the body makes after menopause is oestrone1. Oestradiol is the most prevalent estrogen type in women of reproductive age.

Estrogen in the body

Estrogen functions throughout the body and is a crucial hormone throughout puberty, assisting in the onset of the menstrual cycle and physical changes.Oestrogen is a critical hormone in fertility and has a role in controlling the menstrual cycle as well as maintaining pregnancy.

Throughout the month, estrogen levels in women fluctuate; they are greatest throughout the menstrual cycle and lowest during a woman's period. Ovulation, or the development and release of an egg, is made possible by the generation of oestradiol.

In addition to influencing bone and heart health, estrogen is crucial for brain and mood regulation. Women going through the menopause will have higher cholesterol levels since oestrogen helps regulate cholesterol.

Menopause's Estrogen levels

Estrogen and progesterone levels fluctuate during the perimenopause stage until a woman enters menopause as she ages because her ovarian response slows down with time. This occurs when a lady goes a whole year without having her period. Premenopausal women's typical oestrogen levels range between 45-854 pmol/L. By the time a woman reaches menopause and beyond, the levels are fewer than 100 pmol

Estrogen and progesterone concentrations are balanced throughout a typical cycle. But as women enter their mid-30s to early 40s Both progesterone levels and estrogen production start to decline as a result.

Women may see a shift in their menstrual cycles as a result. They might be heavier or lighter, occur more frequently or less frequently, endure for longer or shorter periods of time, etc. Having missing periods during perimenopause is common. Towards the conclusion of the perimenopause, there is a sudden drop in oestrogen, which is known to cause the menopausal symptoms including hot flushes, vaginal dryness, and memory problems. Periods may be shorter and less frequent in this situation.

Healthy bones and estrogen
Women going through the menopause must take care of their bone health because as oestrogen levels fall, bones become thinner and weaker, increasing the risk of osteoporosis.Between five and Seven years after menopause, women may lose up to one-fifth % of their whole body weight as a result of the declining oestrogen levels, of their bone density.Oestrogen has a significant impact on the health of a woman's bones. As a result, dropping levels will result in worsening bone health.

As a woman ages, maintaining bone health depends on diet and activity. Bone health may be supported by eating a diet high in elements essential for bone health, such as

calcium and magnesium, and by taking a vitamin D supplement. Yoga and other weight-bearing workouts will also help.
Loading the skeleton and staying physically active will assist. Try dancing, walking, and strength training, for instance. Look at the article "Strong, Steady, Straight" on the Royal Osteoporosis Society website to learn how to fight osteoporosis with exercise.

Progesterone
A steroid hormone called progesterone is created by the body during ovulation. Its primary function is to get a woman's body ready for pregnancy.When ovulation takes place, a tiny cluster of cells known as the corpus luteum develops where the ovary delivers the egg. Progesterone production originates in the corpus luteum.

The body gets ready for pregnancy via progesterone. On day 21 of the menstrual cycle, progesterone levels often reach their peak. The corpus luteum dissolves, progesterone levels fall, and a woman gets her period if the egg is not fertilized. The corpus luteum will continue generating progesterone if an egg is fertilized. The placenta replaces the ovaries as the primary source of progesterone a few weeks during pregnancy. The hormone is produced in large quantities by the placenta throughout a typical pregnancy.

Menopause and progesterone
Progesterone acts in opposition to estrogen during the typical menstrual cycle to maintain the proper balance of both hormones. Progesterone takes control in the next phase of the menstrual cycle to prepare the body for pregnancy or until the period starts, whereas estrogen increases in the initial phase to encourage the development of an egg.
However, a woman's menstrual cycle is less predictable during the perimenopause

because her ovaries are less sensitive, and low progesterone levels can also result in bigger menstrual bleeds2. Declining progesterone levels might produce other symptoms including vaginal dryness in addition to alterations in a woman's menstrual cycle. Progesterone contributes to the thickening of the cervical mucus, but when levels decline during the menopause, this can result in dryness of the vagina.

Estrogen is only one component of female hormones. Estrogen to progesterone ratios fluctuate according to a predetermined rhythm during the period cycle. Therefore, physiological changes will arise from the decline in both hormones throughout peri and after menopause, typically at distinct speeds and in a diverse manner. These modifications to hormone rhythms have effects on the body, mind, and soul. Menopause symptoms are brought on by low progesterone levels, which can no longer maintain a healthy balance with oestrogen levels, leading to oestrogen dominance before its own decrease.

Testosterone

As the "male hormone," testosterone is frequently associated more with males than with women. However, a woman's body also depends heavily on testosterone. Women's ovaries and adrenal glands generate testosterone, which helps to maintain proper metabolic function, muscular and bone strength, mood, and cognitive function in addition to desire, sexual excitement, and orgasm in females.

The ovaries and testicles generate 50 percent of all endogenous testosterone. The adrenals create half of it. Around 100-400 mcg of testosterone, or three to four times as much as oestrogen generated in the ovaries, were produced daily by healthy young women.

In actuality, levels fall in half between 20 and 40.Low libido, modifications in mood and cognitive function, and an increased risk of osteoporosis are all consequences of declining testosterone levels. Acne and a rise in facial hair development are potential side effects for post-menopausal women, but genetics also play a significant impact in the likelihood of developing these issues.

Chapter 3

Nutrition In Menopause

Although menopause is a visible event, the menopausal transition may take many years and the health consequences of postmenopausal hypoestrogenism may linger for decades, even after symptoms are no longer apparent. Menopause is connected with increased incidence of obesity, metabolic syndrome, cardiovascular disease, and osteoporosis.

Weight increase is reported among midlife women and has been related to both chronological aging and to the menopausal transition. Recent results from a large population-based cohort in the United

States. confirmed the assumption that weight gain is not simply connected to the menopausal transition, even if the fat mass grows fast in this time. In this context, a population-based research that we did in southern Brazil indicated that sedentariness rather than menopause is related with a two-fold higher risk of overweight/obesity. Therefore, exercise together with calorie restriction should be advocated in all those postmenopausal women with excess weight, for decreases in metabolic and cardiovascular risk..

The capacity to transition from fat utilization during fasting to carbohydrate utilization during hyperinsulinemia is known as metabolic flexibility. Gonadal hormones could govern metabolic flexibility at the level of the mitochondria, influencing how nutrients are turned into energy.

In postmenopausal women, metabolic flexibility declines owing to estrogen loss and more fat accumulates in central depots.

The holistic health care of menopausal women should thus stress lifestyle evaluation and counseling to offset the negative effects of estrogen deprivation on general well-being and limit the risk of metabolic syndrome, osteoporosis, bone fractures, and vascular events. Among the different components of health promotion and lifestyle adaptation to the postmenopausal age, dietary habits are crucial since they affect all women, can be improved, and effect both lifespan and quality of life.

In this narrative review, we shall discuss the current evidence on the association between dietary patterns and clinical endpoints in postmenopausal women, such as body composition, bone mass, and risk markers for cardiovascular disease (CVD), including studies of risk association and/or effects of dietary interventions and thereby providing novel insight into the establishment of optimal dietary guidelines for healthy postmenopausal period.

Dietary Intake

In the menopausal' transition, declining estrogen levels have been connected with loss of lean body mass (LBM) and rise in fat mass. In the longitudinal Study of Women's Health Across the Nation, LBM loss during the menopausal transition averaged 0.5% (a mean annual absolute decline of 0.2 kg), whereas FM grew by 1.7% per year (mean annual absolute rise of 0.45 kg) (mean annual absolute increase of 0.45 kg).

Body composition alterations in this cohort were related with higher risk of coronary heart disease, possibly jeopardizing the woman's health as a whole. In the National Health and Nutrition Examination Survey (NHANES), people with low LBM and high FM had the greatest cardiovascular and overall mortality risk.

Dietary Protein Ageing raises dietary protein needs] because skeletal muscles diminish their capability of triggering protein synthesis in response to anabolic stimuli, potentially owing to insulin resistance. In fact, observational studies have revealed that increased protein consumption is related with higher LBM in postmenopausal women.

In the Women's Health Initiative research, increased protein consumption (1.2 g/kg body weight) was related with a 32% decreased incidence of frailty and improved physical function]. The mean protein consumption related with increased skeletal muscle mass index in postmenopausal women was 1.6 g/kg body weight. but the Institute of Medicine advises for all ages the protein requirement of 0.8 g/kg body weight. Because observational data are unable to distinguish the direction of cause and effect, randomized controlled trials (RCT) have been created to confirm this theory.

A meta-analysis of 36 RCTs involving 1682 individuals found that protein supplementation, from 6 to 78 weeks, did not contribute to increase in LBM in non-frail community-dwelling older persons. The few published interventional trials concentrating on postmenopausal women have revealed that increased protein consumption did not improve LBM growth when compared to recommended dietary allowance (RDA) (RDA).

Indeed, beyond the metabolic and physiological changes of aging that may affect protein metabolism. The present research shows that RDA may be adequate to preserve LBM in older women.Dietary Carbohydrate, Whole Grains, and Glycemic Index The significance of dietary carbohydrate for inducing FM loss has to be understood. In obese patients, a prior comprehensive analysis has found that modest low carbohydrate diet (40% of total calories) was not related with reduction in fat mass.

Recently, a randomized control experiment with 57 women (age 40 ± 3.5 years, BMI 31.1 ± 2.6 kg·m−2) produced comparable findings, with low-carbohydrate-high-fat diets having no greater impact on FM in contrast to a normal diet.

However, certain carbohydrate sources may be advantageous, while others are not, depending at least in part on their fiber level. In an RCT with 81 males and 32 postmenopausal women, the intake of whole grains over six weeks had favorable effects on the resting metabolic rate and stool energy excretion, which affected positively the energy balance.

Indeed, this research offers evidence for dietary guidelines suggesting the use of whole grains instead than refined grains in order to lower adiposity, but there are relatively few interventional studies concentrating on postmenopausal women.

Complementing alternative means of categorizing carbohydrate diets, such as fiber and whole grain content, glycemic index (GI) should also be regarded especially significant in decreasing total body FM and regulating weight.

Eating a meal with high GI stimulates a speedy pancreatic response to the increasing blood glucose levels, with significant insulin production that quickly reduces blood glucose and increases hunger and overeating.

Bone Health

The decline in bone mineral density (BMD) that follows aging is connected to diminishing reproductive hormone. BMD loss increases considerably during the late perimenopause, when menses become more irregular. Several studies have established the necessity of appropriate calcium and vitamin D consumption for improved BMD and prevention..

However, the recommended daily intake of calcium for older individuals varies from 700 mg , while the North American Menopause Society actually advises 1000 to 1500 mg of dietary calcium per day to postmenopausal women . Available data from completed RCTs offered no support for the use of vitamin D or calcium supplementations alone to prevent fractures.

On the other hand, regular treatment with both vitamin D (400–800 IU/day) and calcium (1000–1200 mg/day) was a more promising method.Besides, study of isolated nutrients is not adequate to uncover the intricate interactions between nutrients and non-nutrients found in diet. Therefore, the study of dietary patterns, especially the MD pattern, has been recommended to evaluate the association between diet and BMD. Previous research revealed that higher adherence to the MD is favorably linked with BMD in middle-aged and older persons and in postmenopausal women.

Recent data from an RCT done across five European locations confirm similar conclusions from observational research. In this experiment, an MD-like diet recommended for one year and accompanied by personalized guidance and supply of the essential items generated a substantial reduction in the rate of BMD loss among patients with osteoporosis, compared to a group that got simply informational leaflets.

Cardiovascular Risk

The estrogens released by the ovaries throughout the reproductive phase exhibit protective effects on vascular endothelial function as well as on lipid metabolism. After menopause, the relative estrogen shortage leads to elevate vascular tone via both endocrine and autonomic pathways that culminate decreased nitric oxide reliant vasodilation.

Postmenopausal women had two to three times greater prevalence of metabolic syndrome, compared to same aged premenopausal women. The modifications in cardiovascular risk begin during the perimenopause phase.

Menopause transition resulted in lipid profile modifications, with a 10–15% increased LDL-cholesterol and triglyceride levels and slightly reduced HDL cholesterol levels.This phase also contributes for an increase in BMI and abdominal adiposity, with postmenopausal women exhibiting roughly five times the risk of central obesity compared to premenopausal women.. The prevalence of central obesity has been related with reduced heart rate variability, another indication of subclinical CVD

Scientific organizations propose the following healthy food pattern to lower the risk of major chronic illnesses and promote overall wellness. protein sources mostly from plants, nuts, fish, or other sources of omega-3 fatty acids; fat predominantly from unsaturated plant sources; carbs primarily from whole grains; at least five servings of fruits and vegetables per day; and moderate dairy intake as an option.

Low-energy diet is also recommended for postmenopausal women to prevent metabolic alterations. In a cross-sectional study of 4984 women aged 30–79 years, three dietary patterns (Western, healthy, and traditional) were identified. In a stratified analysis by menopausal status, the inverse association of the healthy dietary pattern (characterized by high factor loadings with green-yellow vegetables, healthy-protein foods, seaweeds, and bonefish) and metabolic syndrome was statistically significant only among postmenopausal women.
In analyzing each component of metabolic syndrome, the healthy eating pattern was

shown to be protective for blood pressure and triglyceride levels among premenopausal women and for obesity and HDL-cholesterol levels among postmenopausal women.

A decline in energy expenditure throughout midlife may potentially produce obesity during menopause. According to a four-year follow-up research, the decline in physical activity started two years before menopause. Aging resulted in increased subcutaneous abdominal fat over time to all women, however, only those who turned postmenopausal experienced a considerable rise in visceral abdominal fat. During the menopausal transition there is a propensity to weight gain accompanied by an increase in central fat distribution that persists throughout the post-menopause.

For postmenopausal women, sedentary lifestyle and a diet with carbohydrate consumption accounting for more than 55%

of total calories correlate to greater cardiovascular risk, according to high sensitivity C-reactive protein levels.

Low-fat diets may lead to greater improvement in LDL cholesterol levels, whereas low-carbohydrate diets may result in greater improvement in triglyceride and HDL cholesterol levels;\sMediterranean diet is associated with a small but significant decrease in blood pressure and reduced CVD risk of among different female cohorts, although more evidence is required for these outcomes in postmenopausal women.

Chapter 4

Suggested Diet Plan For Menopause

When you're navigating the often complex route of menopause, you may need all the aid you can get. Hot flashes, nocturnal sweats, mood swings, and sexual dysfunction may really take a toll. One simple, natural approach you may attempt to relieve some of these menopausal symptoms is to include these eight kinds of foods to your meals.

Although managing menopause might seem like you're on an emotional roller coaster, the ride could feel a bit easier if you make a few easy dietary modifications.Some risk factors and symptoms related with aging and menopause can't be modified. But excellent eating may help avoid or lessen some illnesses that may emerge during and after menopause. During menopause, consume a variety of meals to receive all the nutrients you need.

- Soy Milk, Soy Beans, Edamame, Miso, Tofu, Tempeh

A tiny research called the WAVS experiment looked at postmenopausal women who experienced two or more hot flashes a day. Thirty-eight women were placed into two groups: One group got a soy-rich, low-fat vegan diet, which comprised 1/2 cup of cooked soybeans per day; the other did not.

The findings, published in July 2021 in Menopause, indicated that overall hot flashes dropped by 79 percent and moderate to severe hot flashes fell by 84 percent in the soy foods group, compared with 49 percent and 42 percent, respectively, in the control group. After the trial completed, 59 percent of soy group participants indicated that they no longer suffered moderate or severe hot flashes.

- Steel-Cut Oats, Barley, Wheat, Brown Rice, Bulgur, Popcorn, Millet

Whole grains provide a plethora of nutrients, according to the Harvard T.H. Chan School of Public Health, including B vitamins and fiber. B vitamins are crucial for the neurological system and mood, while fiber helps keep you regular. Research also showed that eating whole grains instead of processed grains might lessen your risk of cardiovascular disease. " Read food labels. Choose foods that feature 100 percent whole grains or 100 percent whole wheat as the first ingredient on the label.

- Parsley, Sage, Rosemary, and Thyme (plus Oregano, Basil, and Mint) (and Oregano, Basil, and Mint)

Hot flashes may be induced by consuming spicy foods, among other causes, writes the Cleveland Clinic. But this doesn't mean you have to confine yourself to bland dishes. If you want to add flavor, try mild spices and seasonings, such as basil, bay leaf, cardamom, Chinese five spice mix, cinnamon, coriander, lemon balm, mint, oregano, rosemary, sage, thyme, and parsley. "These all provide exquisite flavors but without producing a heat flash.

- Chocolate

Okay, before you go shotgunning Lindt truffles, there are some boundaries to this. A small study published in the July 2021 issue of The FASEB Journal reports that among 19 postmenopausal women, eating a concentrated amount of milk chocolate during morning or nighttime (100 grams of chocolate daily) did not lead to weight gain, and a high intake of chocolate during the morning hours helped burn fat and reduce blood glucose levels.

A restricted research published in July 2020 in the European Journal of Preventive Cardiology proposes that consuming any sort of chocolate more than once weekly may lower the incidence of cardiovascular events by 8 percent. If you have an option, go for dark chocolate. According to the Harvard T.H. Chan School of Public Health, it includes heart-healthy flavanols that help decrease blood pressure; other studies have indicated a correlation between ingesting 6 grams of dark chocolate per day and a lower risk of heart disease.

- Fruits and vegetables

Many women are disturbed by weight gain during menopause. Besides also having high water content, fruits and vegetables that are rich in fiber might help you feel full while ingesting less calories, according to the Mayo Clinic. Let fruits and vegetables take up half of the real estate on your plate at mealtimes and even during snack time.

Another symptom wrinkle may be addressed by eating mangos, according to a study published in November 2020 in the journal Nutrients (the study was financed by the Mango Board and done by academics at the University of California in Davis) (the study was supported by the Mango Board and conducted by researchers at the University of California in Davis). In this research, postmenopausal women who swallowed 1/3 cup of Ataulfo mangoes four times a week observed a 23 percent drop in deep wrinkles after two months.

If consumed regularly, prunes, according to study published in May 2021 in the Journal of Medicinal Food, enhance risk factors for cardiovascular disease, including enhancing

antioxidant capacity and lowering inflammation among healthy, postmenopausal women.
entire grains or 100 percent whole wheat as the first component on the label.

- Water

Getting adequate H20 may relieve a range of symptoms: lowering vaginal dryness, perhaps enhancing the skin's look, and minimizing bloat by moving fiber along. Signs of dehydration include thirst, muscular cramps, dry skin, weariness, and disorientation. "There is no one-size-fits-all advice for daily allowance. Your greatest guide is to examine your pee. If you are adequately hydrated, it will be light yellow. If it is a deep yellow, you need to start drinking more.

You may satisfy your water requirements with water-rich meals such as watermelon, strawberries, and soups. Stay away from alcohol, which may be dehydrating. Experiment with various tastes: Add a lemon wedge, a dash of mint, or cucumber slices. You may enjoy it at various temperatures. Finally, make things simple on yourself by always having a full water bottle available.

- Salmon, Herring, Sardines, Trout, Mackerel

Essential fatty acids found in oily fish, particularly omega-3s, have been shown to help promote heart health, notes the American Heart Association. The risk of heart disease rises with women, particularly as they age, therefore these good fats are really essential. Omega-3s may also help alleviate mood problems. Low-Fat Yogurt, Milk, and Cheese, Plus Dark, Leafy Greens and Calcium-Fortified Products Like Almond Milk, Cereals, and Orange Juice.

Due to hormonal changes, women undergo significant bone loss during menopause, sometimes leading to postmenopausal osteoporosis. According to the North American Menopause Society, 1 in 2 women over age 50 will have an osteoporosis-related fracture in her lifetime.

Protect your bones by receiving adequate calcium from dairy and calcium-fortified products. According to the Mayo Clinic, women age 19 to 50 should strive for 1,000 milligrams (mg) a day while women 51 and beyond should obtain 1,200 mg a day. Your body requires vitamin D to absorb calcium, says the National Institutes of Health (NIH) (NIH). Some vitamin D sources include fatty foods like salmon, egg yolks, and simple sun exposure, according to the NIH

- Cut down on high-fat meals.

Fat should give 25% to 35% or less of your total daily calories. Also, restrict saturated fat to less than 7% of your total daily calories. Saturated fat elevates cholesterol and enhances your risk for heart disease. It's found in fatty foods, full milk, ice cream, and cheese. Limit cholesterol to 300 mg or less per day. And watch out for trans fats, found in vegetable oils, many baked goods, and some margarine. Trans fat also raises cholesterol and increases your risk for heart disease.

- Use sugar and salt in moderation.

Too much salt in the diet is connected to high blood pressure. Also, go light on smoked, salt-cured, and charbroiled meals — these foods contain high amounts of nitrates, which have been related to cancer.

Chapter 5

The Good In Menopause

The concept of menopause normally draws to mind an assortment of undesirable symptoms, hot flashes, vaginal dryness, mood swings, receding hair, sleep issues. The list is extensive and disappointing. But menopause may have a beneficial influence on your life as well; for one thing, not all bodily changes induced by lower female hormone levels are harmful.

For another, many of the emotional and social shifts might really be stimulating. Read on to find out what many women have already discovered: In many respects, menopause may be a welcome transition.

- No more periods

Menopause signifies the end of the monthly cycle, which for many women is a reason for joy in itself. It means no more fiddling with tampons or pads, no more fear about leaking, and no more period cramps. And after the perimenopausal years, when periods typically become erratic and bleeding may be severe, it puts an end to the guessing game of when your period is going to start or cease. "Some women are even restricted to their houses on days when bleeding is excessive. For them, menopause may be tremendously freeing.

- Goodbye to PMS

In the week or two before your period, premenstrual syndrome (PMS) may induce a number of physical and mental symptoms, ranging from breast soreness and headache pain to food cravings and irritability. PMS is fairly common: According to the American College of Obstetricians and Gynecologists, at least 85 percent of all menstrual women suffer one symptom or more each month. In perimenopause, PMS may temporarily worsen as estrogen levels increase and decrease. All the better, therefore, to have PMS vanish after menopause.

"Perimenopause entails a lot of years of a really hard hormonal ride, so there's no doubt, especially for women who have experienced mood problems around these hormonal fluxes, that menopause may be a 'Ahhhh!' sort of period,"

- Sex Without Pregnancy Worries

Women in menopause may enjoy sex without having to fret about a potential pregnancy. This makes a major impact, according to the Investigation of Women's Health Across the Nation, a multisite, longitudinal study of the physical and psychological changes women encounter in midlife, including menopause. "Among American women of diverse ethnic groups, sex without worrying about pregnancy was widely identified as one of the perks of menopause," says Nanette Santoro, MD, professor and head of Reproductive Endocrinology at Albert Einstein College of Medicine in New York. Some women even discover that, since they no longer have to worry about the unplanned consequence of sex, they may actually enjoy it more after they enter menopause.

● The End of Hormonal Headaches
Women are impacted by headaches three times more commonly than males, according to the National Headache Foundation. About 70 percent of these women get menstrual migraines, headaches that correlate with ovulation and menstruation. Like other migraines, these headaches involve throbbing pain on one side of the head, occasionally accompanied by nausea, vomiting, and light- or sound-sensitivity. In a normal monthly cycle, changing amounts of the hormones estrogen and progesterone may produce menstrual migraines. But after menopause, levels of estrogen and progesterone reduce, and frequently the frequency of hormonal headaches falls too. "Headaches might temporarily intensify during the tumultuous hormone changes associated with

perimenopause, but migraine patients can look forward to an improvement after they are through the menopausal transition.

- Uterine Fibroids Shrink

Many women entering their 50s acquire fibroids, uterine tumors that are nearly often benign. Fibroids develop when estrogen levels in the body are high – during pregnancy, when levels of estrogen and progesterone rise, and in perimenopause, when estrogen levels may range from low to high. If fibroid symptoms, including discomfort, heavy menstrual blood, and strain on the bladder are severe, physicians may consider surgery. Fortunately, fibroids generally cease growing or shrink when women approach menopause and estrogen levels fall. For women who have been documenting fibroid development hoping to avoid surgery, or for those who have heavy periods owing to fibroids, menopause is welcome.